COMPLEMENTARY AND ALTERNATIVE
THERAPIES FOR PAIN.

Your Guide to over 50 treatments for pain relief.

By
Barbara McLullich

INTRODUCTION.

Barbara McLullich was born in Manchester, has lived in Cheshire and Spain, and now lives in Nottinghamshire with her husband. She has two children, living in Australia and Brighton.

After successfully running her own businesses for several years, Barbara had to call a halt to commerce when a number of surgical processes to alleviate her back pain failed to cure the problem. Driven by her own relentless energy, she resolved to write about her experiences with pain, and so created an award-winning blog which deals comprehensively with the subject, at www.backpain.blog.co.uk

This book has been assembled and written by Barbara, with a view to providing a mainly objective but often personal view of the plethora of alternative approaches to pain relief available in the UK today. It does not attempt to offer any scientific or biological assessment of each treatment, nor purport to differentiate between the relative success or failure of each process. The book simply serves as an anthology of a selection of well-known and currently employed techniques, available either through the National Health Service (NHS) or from various private practitioners across the country, with some additional studies from the USA used for supplementary information.

Barbara has written a number of online books and blogs daily on the subject of back and neck pain, herself having suffered for most of her adult life with the debilitating challenges severe spinal discomfort can bring. Many of the treatments here she has tried herself and has attempted in the book to provide an objective view of each alternative, whether or not she has personally utilised it and whether or not it has been of any benefit to her. Barbara is not medically qualified, but suggests that with the amount of treatment and the variety of attempts to cure her back and neck problems employed over the last 30 years by all kinds of practitioners, from neurosurgeons to masseuses, she has a breadth of experience that would be hard to match. Her book intentionally steers clear of providing medical evaluations, but attempts to put the essence of the treatment in layman's language and give further reading on each of the 56 therapies she has selected here.

The list in her own words, is *"by no means exhaustive"* but provides a genuine attempt to offer information to those who may be reaching desperation in their quest to find a solution to chronic spinal pain.

CONTENTS.

CHAPTER ONE:
WHAT ARE COMPLEMENTARY THERAPIES?

A complementary therapy is one that can be used in addition to, or instead of, conventional Western medicine.

Of course, you can get a few treatments on the NHS via pain clinics: the waiting list is long but well worth getting on to. Some of the treatments available on the NHS are homoeopathy, herbal medicine, reflexology, acupuncture, nutrition, shiatsu massage and aromatherapy. You can also get some of these treatments from your nearest training college for a quarter of the price charged by normal salons.

Other treatments available at colleges, include pedicures, manicures and waxes, treatments I can no longer do myself.

You can also join some of the discount companies online that offer reductions in your area for a number of things, including include spas and beauty treatments.

Our doctors and health services are overstretched as it is, whereas most alternative practitioners have time to explore our problems in a bit more depth.

They should never be considered as a replacement for conventional medicine, but the two can certainly go hand in hand. Some treatments are far from 'new', with documentation on aromatherapy dating back 5000 years.

With so many people now trying out complementary and natural remedies, it's important   you find out that they are fully-qualified. The Complementary and Natural Healthcare Council's register - http://www.cnhc.org.uk/ - has practitioners who meet the standards of proficiency for their field. They must also hold professional indemnity insurance, have no criminal record and agree to abide by a code of conduct.

CHAPTER TWO:
THE ALEXANDER TECHNIQUE.

The Alexander Technique was originally developed by F. Matthias Alexander (1869-1955), an actor and teacher who originally developed it as a method of vocal training for singers and actors.

He could see that successful vocal training needed a good breathing technique. His methods made such a difference to their breathing that doctors started referring patients with respiratory problems for an Alexander Technique session.

The process aims to change movement habits in everyday activities, helping people with chronic back pain, excessive stress and injury, by using simple and practical methods of balance in the body to release unnecessary tension.

It's a method of teaching improved posture, too, which is beneficial for easing back pain, and helps facilitate movement.

It is said that posture problems and muscle tension are quite often the reason for some of your pain. The technique is safe for people of all ages and in fact, many elderly people and pregnant women benefit from this treatment. It helps millions of people across the world with back, neck and joint pain, muscle tension and stiffness, poor posture, breathing and vocal problems, and anxiety and stress related conditions.

This website has a list of UK teachers of the Alexander Technique - http://www.alexandertechnique.com/teacher/gb/ - but there is no legal requirement for certification necessary to teach it. A good book on the subject is entitled *'How to Stand, How to Move, How to Live : Learning the Alexander Technique to Explore Your Mind Body Connection and Achieve self Mastery'* by Missy Vineyard.

The NHS held a study on the technique which involved over 500 people with chronic back pain. It found that people who received one-to-one instruction of the Alexander Technique, along with exercise, had reduced back pain. Details on the Alexander Technique are also available on the NHS website - http://www.nhs.uk/conditions/alexander-technique/Pages/Introduction.aspx

CHAPTER THREE:
AROMATHERAPY.

According to Mary Margaret Chappell in a recent article in 'Arthritis Today', recent studies *"corroborate the use of aromatherapy for pain relief"*.

Apparently *"Aromatherapy is effective because it works directly on the amygdala, the brain's emotional centre,"* says Mehmet Oz MD, professor of surgery at Columbia University Medical Centre in New York City.

"This has important consequences because the thinking part of the brain can't inhibit the effects of the scent, meaning you feel them instantaneously".

It is a method of healing using highly concentrated plant oils called 'essential oils' that are often highly aromatic and are extracted from plants.

Alan Hirsch MD, neurologist at the Smell and Taste Treatment and Research Foundation in Chicago, believes you don't have to limit yourself to essential oils. Limiting the length of your exposure to certain scents however, will ensure they remain effective.

"Short-term exposure is key because people stop responding to scents after a few minutes".

When you inhale essential oil molecules, messages are transmitted to the limbic system, and affect heart rate, stress levels, blood pressure, breathing, memory and the immune system. The International Federation of Aromatherapists - http://www.ifaroma.org/us/home/ - are the first and largest governing body in Clinical and Holistic Aromatherapy. They have experience and experts who can offer excellence in Aromatherapy and the Science of Essential Oils. They have pioneered and safeguarded standards of practice of Aromatherapy since 1985 and introduced aromatherapy into NHS Hospitals, Hospices and Care Professions. They have a list of IFA therapists from around the world to help you find an approved therapist.

A good book on the subject is *'The Encyclopaedia of Essential Oils: The Complete Guide to the use of aromatic oils in aromatherapy, herbalism, health and well being'*, by Julia Lawless.

On a personal note, Aromatherapy was the first type of alternative therapy that I had after my second surgery. The hospital I was staying in employed a lady who gave the treatment either while you were in hospital or you could have private treatment. She definitely had healing hands as far as I was concerned and, although I am quite sure some of the relief was placebo-effect, I still had regular treatments with her for a short pain-free time.

CHAPTER FOUR:
AURICULAR THERAPY.

Auricular therapy is a method of healing by stimulating different acupressure points on the surface of the outer ear. These areas are pricked with small, sterile, disposable needles in order to help many complaints. In auricular acupuncture, the ear is seen as a micro system of the body.

Auricular therapists believe that there are over 200 points on the ear that are connected to a particular organ, tissue or part of the body. So, if something is out of sync, its corresponding point on the ear may be sensitive or tender to touch and pressure, or a mark, spot or lump can be visible.

Stimulation of the ear is then carried out by means of acupuncture needles, minute electric currents or a laser beam.

An auricular acupuncture session involves placing 5 or 6 small, sterile, disposable needles in each ear. The needles are placed in acupoints corresponding to the area to be treated, so they may place a needle in the neck point if you were suffering from pain in that area.

It is claimed that the therapy can be helpful for various chronic conditions including rheumatism and arthritis.

The actual practice of manipulating needles in the ear to cure diseases is not a new therapy, but a very ancient one. It has been used for many hundreds of years in some Eastern and Mediterranean countries and in China and is also now becoming popular in the UK.

A good book on the therapy is '*Handbook to Chinese Auricular Therapy*' by Ken Chen and Yongqiang Cui and there is an excellent website on the therapy at - http://www.auricularacupuncture.org.uk/saac/?p=find

CHAPTER FIVE:
ACUPUNCTURE THERAPY.

Acupuncture is now available for lower back pain on the NHS. NICE has recommended that acupuncture be made available on the NHS for anyone suffering from chronic low back pain.

A UK trial showed patients who received ten acupuncture sessions were far more likely to be pain-free after two years than those who didn't.

An American study saw 60% of back pain sufferers experience a significant improvement after acupuncture.

The word "acupuncture" means "needle piercing". It is a traditional Chinese medical treatment using very fine needles, which are inserted into the skin at any of the 800 specially-designated points. It originated from a Dutch physician, William Ten Rhyne, who had been living in Japan during the latter part of the 17th century and it was he who introduced it to Europe.

It works by manipulating the body's energy flow, or Chi, to help the body to balance and heal itself.

Legend has it that acupuncture was developed when it was seen that soldiers who recovered from arrow wounds were sometimes also healed of other diseases from which they were suffering.

I am a true believer in acupuncture and regularly have this for not only my lower back pain but also my neck pain, and have seriously thought about learning the techniques so that I could apply the needles to myself.

There are a number of good sites on this therapy, but a good starter is - http://www.acupuncture.org.uk - and an excellent book is *'The Acupuncture Handbook – How acupuncture works and how it can help you'*, by Angela Hicks.

CHAPTER SIX:
ACUPRESSURE THERAPY.

Acupressure is an ancient Chinese healing method which has been around for over 3000 years, and which works on the 'meridians' of your body, and is similar to acupuncture but without the needles.

'Meridians' are the pathways of the positive and negative energy power, which carry on some of the communication between the various parts of our body. They are electro-magnetic in character and consist of small palpable spots, which can be located by hand.

There are 500 points and are classified as ying or yang on the basis of the direction in which they flow on the surface of the body.

In a healthy body, the 'Chi' flows freely and evenly through the meridians but if there is illness or disease in the body then the 'Chi' gets blocked.

To release the blocked 'Chi', acupressure is used to work on key pressure points, using thumbs similar to needles in Acupuncture. When these triggers are pressed, they release muscular tension, promote blood circulation and increase the flow of energy.

Acupressure.com - http://www.acupressure.com/ - is a website totally dedicated to acupressure where you can find out how to teach yourself administration of this treatment.

There is also a lot of information, videos, products, charts and everything you need to know about this therapy.

Also check out this book - 'Acupressure. How to cure common ailments the natural way', by Michael Reed Gach.

CHAPTER SEVEN:
BOWEN TECHNIQUE.

The Bowen Technique has now joined the group of complementary therapies to be recognised by the Complementary and Natural Healthcare Council (CNHC), which provides an independent national standard of excellence.

The CNHC is the only voluntary regulatory body for complementary healthcare to have official backing from the government. Its key function is to enhance public protection by setting standards for registration with CNHC.

The BOWEN technique was developed in the 1960's and 1970's, by Thomas Ambrose Bowen, an osteopath from Australia.

It has been called 'miraculous' and is a soft tissue remedial therapy that involves the therapist using fingers and thumbs to move over muscle, ligament, tendons and fascia, in various parts of the body.

The main feature of the Bowen Technique is that between each set of moves, the therapist leaves the patient to rest for a short while to allow the body the opportunity to create a decision about what action needs to be taken in response to the moves given (sounds _so_ relaxing).

It's a gentle, non-invasive, relaxing therapy to help free the body to return to its natural balance and healing.

My choice of book on this therapy is _'The Bowen Technique'_, by Julian Baker.

The Bowen Therapy Professional Association - http://www.bowen-therapy.co/ - is an independent organisation of Bowen Therapists run by Bowen Therapists. The website is full of information on the Bowen Technique and has a list of practitioners.

CHAPTER EIGHT:
BIBLIOTHERAPY.

Have you ever heard of a Bibliotherapist?

Well, neither had I until I read an article about them.

Basically, a Bibliotherapist is a reading therapist who works out a person's reading habits, ambitions and stage in their life, and then draws up a prescription of books for the client to read.

It's a way of using books to aid people in solving the issues that they may be facing at a particular time. It can also be combined with writing therapy and has been known to help treat depression.

They have found that some people suffering from chronic pain enjoyed some pain relief once they understood their condition, by reading the correct publication about it.

To find out lots more about it, go to The School of Life website - http://www.theschooloflife.com/Bibliotherapy

CHAPTER NINE:
BALNEOTHERAPY.

Balneotherapy is one of the oldest therapies for pain relief.

The term 'balneo' comes from the Latin word, *balneum*, meaning bath.

Balneotherapy is a form of hydrotherapy which involves bathing in mineral water or warm water. A study compared bathing in mineral water to plain tap water in 60 people with lower back pain and Fibromyalgia. They found that mineral water containing sulphur was superior in reducing pain and improving mobility, compared with tap water.

In the journal 'Rheumatology', a systematic review and meta-analysis assessed spa therapy and balneotherapy, and found that they definitely helped with lower back pain.

CHAPTER TEN:
CRYSTAL HEALING.

Crystals are decorative, fascinating gemstones and come in all shapes and sizes. They have magical powers and properties and they generate, store, regulate, transmit and transform energy.

It is a holistic therapy that has been used since ancient times for physical healing. So, if you were deficient in a specific type of energy, you were given a specific stone to wear.

Everything in the universe is made up of some sort of energy. The chair you sit on, the cup you drink out of. When a person's mind or body is in disharmony through unsettled thoughts or disease, a crystal placed on or near the person is supposed to transform the person to a state of balance and harmony.

By putting out good vibes, they harmonise the atmosphere and transmit good energy. This energy means that crystals can be used for certain tasks, such as directing healing energy to a specific point that may have a blockage.

While you wear your crystal as jewellery or in a pouch, the crystal vibrations work continuously on your imbalances. They say it is important to keep the crystal on you all the time (24hrs a day) for at least 21 days in order for the cleansing process to be initiated.

It can take up to three to four months or longer to harmonise your body and if you carry on wearing the stones or crystals after that period, it is believed that you will achieve continuous stability.

The Therapy Directory - http://www.therapy-directory.org.uk/articles/crystal-therapy.html - explains in great detail about crystal therapy and can help you find a crystal therapist near you.

There is also a very good book on this type of healing called 'The Complete Guide to Crystal Healing : Energy Medicine for Mind, Body and Spirit by Philip Permutt.

Philip, who is also a Reiki Master, has written other books and articles on this subject and writes Crystal Clinic, a monthly column for Take a Break's Fate and Fortune magazine.

His articles have also been published in Positive Health, Prediction, Natural Health, Spirit and Destiny, Paradigm Shift and High Spirit Magazines. He has also written booklets for several of Paradise Music's CD releases and has compiled and published The Dawning (magazine).

CHAPTER ELEVEN:
CHIROPRACTIC CARE.

Chiropractic care is a safe and generally accepted method of treating spinal pain.

The word 'chiropractic' originates from two Greek words - 'kheir,' which means 'hand' and 'praktikos', which means 'practical'.

A healer called Daniel Palmer (1845-1913), found he was able to cure a man's deafness that had occurred when he bent down and felt a bone click. When he examined him, Palmer found that some bones of the man's spine had become displaced. After successful manipulation treatment from Palmer, the man regained his hearing.

This discipline has a wide variety of techniques that aim to correct dysfunctions that can cause irregularities in the spinal structure and its movement.

Of course, the discipline does not claim to be the best solution for spinal pain like sciatica or lower back pain. Physicians actually recommend chiropractic treatments as a form of alternative medicine, rather than an initial option for pain relief.

Chiropractors use a technique they call "spinal manipulation" for treating the affected area. Spinal manipulation is a combination of dynamic but controlled methods of force that are meant to make the joints move past their normal range of movement without rupturing or dislocating them.

Chiropractors are completely different from massage therapists, as the chiropractor focuses on joints and the spine.

I was personally under the care of a Chiropractor for a number of years, and each time my back went out, he would get me straight again. He kept me away from the operating table for many years.

The British Chiropractic Association site - http://www.chiropractic-uk.co.uk/ - has everything you need to know about Chiropractic care and where to find a professional Chiropractor.

Another good book is 'The Chiropractor's Health Book: Simple Natural Exercises for Relieving Stress', by Leonard McGill.

CHAPTER TWELVE:
COGNITIVE BEHAVIOURAL THERAPY.

Cognitive Therapy was first developed by a medical doctor, psychiatrist and psychoanalyst called Aaron Beck, from America. He put it together in the middle of the 1960's after being certain that he was not getting enough improvement with his patients through analysis.

Cognitive therapy is all about learning how our thoughts create our moods. By using Cognitive therapy we can recognise and reassess these patterns of negative thoughts and replace them with positive thoughts. Basically, it aims to help you manage your problems by changing how you think and act.

Chronic pain can soon make you feel depressed and cognitive therapy can help a depressed person to recognise which life problems are critical, and which are minor. By talking about your problems it can help you to change how you think (cognitive) and what you do (behaviour) which can help you feel better about life. Cognitive Therapy is not going to take the pain away but helps you to deal with the situation which is making you unhappy and depressed. It is so well recognised now, that it is available on the NHS, and a well-known therapy for many different health problems, including chronic pain and other chronic illnesses. This is because physical health problems can affect people's moods and their lives in so many different and distressing ways.

Cognitive behavioural therapy (CBT) is a type of therapy that aims to help you manage your problems by changing how you think and act, and showing people how to recognise and change unhelpful ways of thinking and behaving. This allows them to be less affected by unhelpful moods and to enjoy life more, even if they still have pain. At its simplest, it is a technique for helping people replace habitual negative thinking with positive thinking, by getting them to see the glass as half full not half empty.
CBT encourages you to talk about:
• how you think about yourself, the world and other people
• how what you do affects your thoughts and feelings
By talking about these things, CBT can help you to change how you think ('cognitive') and what you do ('behaviour'), which can help you feel better about life. It's now available on the NHS and involves weekly or fortnightly sessions with a therapist. The number of sessions required varies greatly depending on your problems and objectives, with treatment usually lasting from six weeks to six months. One patient said, '*I was able to move forward and learn to cope and accept my pain. They taught me how to pace myself better and that in turn meant I was able to laugh again a bit more often, instead of just thinking about my pain all the time*'.

Cognitive Behavioural Therapy for Dummies is an excellent book from Amazon written by Rhena Branch and Rob Wilson. It includes tips on establishing ten healthy attitudes for living as well as ten ways to lighten up.

To find a registered therapist, check - http://www.cbtregisteruk.com/Default.aspx

CHAPTER THIRTEEN:
CUPPING THERAPY.

Cupping therapy is given by using glass cups to create localised partial vacuums. It's an ancient Chinese therapy, found in records dating back 3500 years, and involves using heat inside glass or bamboo cups. This draws up the underlying tissues and causes the blood to form in the area and help the healing process there.

Like other forms of Chinese treatments, they believe in the fact that if the 'Meridians' are blocked in your body, then it makes it difficult for healing to take place. They call Meridians 'Qi' (chi) which are pathways in the body that give you energy for life. There are five meridians on your back, which when opened, allow the energy to travel the whole length of the body. It has even been said that cupping is probably the best way of opening those meridians.

Another healing aspect of cupping therapy is through the release of toxins in your body. Cupping is the best deep tissue massage available and is a very safe therapy to have. It activates the lymphatic systems, clearing colon blockages, arteries and capillaries.

Some of the conditions cupping therapy can be used to treat include constipation, IBS, diarrhoea, headaches, back pain, arthritis, fatigue, sciatica, skin problems, Fibromyalgia, period cramps, weight problems and more. It works by reducing the pain we feel in our bodies.

It involves the use of a warmed cup, which is placed upside down on a specific acupuncture point. This then creates a vacuum to draw the blood and energy to that point.

I had a number of cupping therapy treatments in a Physiotherapy department of the NHS. To be truthful, this therapy did not help me in any way, but that is not to say that it will not help others, otherwise it would not be available on the NHS.

There is a cupping therapy association - http://www.cuppingtherapy.org/ - which is dedicated to helping you in finding out details, practitioners and testimonials.

CHAPTER FOURTEEN:
CRANIOSACRAL THERAPY.

Craniosacral therapy is an alternative medicine therapy, which is an exceptionally gentle yet extremely powerful form of treatment, used by many therapists. It is non-invasive and focuses on restoring our body's natural self-healing mechanisms. It was developed from the work of an American Osteopath, Dr William Sutherland in the early 1990's.

It can be used for several conditions including neck and back pain as well as Fibromyalgia. This type of treatment can be very effective in treating back problems as its aim is to let your body treat itself, until you can feel the pain go away and feel relaxed.

Patients are usually asked to lie down fully-clothed on a treatment couch. A craniosacral therapist will then place their hands lightly on various areas of your body, which allows them to tune into what they call the 'craniosacral rhythm'. They then gently work with the spine and skull and its cranial sutures, diaphragms and fascia, which should then help ease restrictions in nerve passages.

The first thing you will notice is a deep sense of relaxation which you should feel throughout the treatment and will last throughout the session. As it is such a gentle therapy, it is suitable for babies, children and the elderly.

They say everyone can benefit from craniosacral therapy including babies as it focuses on restoring our body's natural self-healing mechanisms, which then encourages the body to re-establish its own good health.

Treatment can aid almost any condition, raising vitality and improving the body's capacity for self repair.

A good website to start at is - www.craniosacral.co.uk - which gives you lots of information on the treatment and links to therapists in your area.

There is also a good book available called *'Craniosacral Therapy'*, by John Upledger and Jon Vredevoogd.

CHAPTER FIFTEEN:
ERICKSONIA THERAPY.

Milton H. Erickson MD, an American (1901-1980), is considered to be the father of modern hypnotherapy. He was born into a poor farming community and didn't speak until he was four and was later found to have severe dyslexia, and to be tone deaf and colour blind.

At 17 he had his first attack of Polio where he went into a coma. When he awoke 3 days later, he found himself completely paralysed, unable to move, except for his eyes, and barely able to speak. Over the next two years, he taught himself to walk again and thus one of the hallmarks of hypnotherapy was born. Despite his problems, Erickson went on to qualify as a medical doctor and psychiatrist.

Much later, when in his Fifties, his polio came back a second time, characterised by pain and muscle weakness caused by the chronic over-use of partially paralysed muscles. This time he had to use a wheelchair, and suffered chronic pain, which he controlled with self-hypnosis. With this he was able to turn it into a learning opportunity and he became very good at treating other people's pain with hypnosis.

He hypnotised more than 30,000 people in the course of his career and wrote the entries on hypnosis for 3 encyclopaedias, including the Britannica (1954-1973) and Colliers Encyclopaedia (1952-1962). He published more than 300 scientific papers, has had more than 100 books written about him and there are more than 110 institutes promoting his Ericksonian Therapy worldwide.

The Erickson Foundation website - http://erickson-foundation.org/ - has lots to offer from training to conferences or just details on the therapy. There are too many books on the subject to even list, but one that caught my eye is called 'Speak Ericksonian' by Richard Nongard.

His book holds the key to the Ericksonian approach to hypnotherapy. It will teach you how to tap into the resources Milton Erickson left in his writings, case studies and books. It also provides scripts, resources, and a clear understanding of what Ericksonian hypnotherapy is all about.

CHAPTER SIXTEEN:
EFT THERAPY.

EFT Therapy is a method based on the discovery that emotional trauma contributes greatly to disease. It's a ground-breaking tool for releasing emotional blocks and healing for phobias, trauma, pain and more.

Studies have shown that EFT can help to reduce the emotional impact of memories and incidents that trigger emotional distress. Once that is removed, then the body can often rebalance itself, which then has a knock-on effect to accelerate healing.

Eastern health practices have been based on the fact that the energies that circulate throughout our bodies are vital to our health. Interrupting these energies can result in pain and disease. This has been their concept for over 5000 years. Therefore, it is no surprise that repairing any disruption in your energy channels can lead to symptom and pain relief.

Wikipedia describes it as a *'form of alternative psychotherapy that purports to manipulate the body's energy field by tapping on acupuncture points'*.

Some call EFT 'a new acupuncture without the needles' and 'energy psychology'.

Success rates for EFT are not 100% but it certainly has a high success rate for some.

A brilliant book on this subject is *' Transform Your Beliefs. Transform Your Life : EFT Tapping Using Matrix Reimprinting',* by Karl Dawson and Kate Marillat.

For more details on EFT and it's practitioners head to the website - http://eft.mercola.com/

CHAPTER SEVENTEEN:
FELDENKRAIS THERAPY.

Feldenkrais Therapy is an educational programme that enhances the communication between your body and your brain. It accentuates personal awareness of your body's mobility patterns and uses movement and structural training. The movements are slow and gentle, and the focus is on correcting posture.

It is named after its originator, Moshe Feldenkrais (1904-1984), an engineer and physicist as well as a Judo teacher.

The benefits of this therapy include relief from tension and muscular pain, easier breathing, greater relaxation, improved performance in sport, dance music and drama and increased vitality.

By heightening our awareness of our movement, breathing and posture, the Feldenkrais Therapy will bring us closer to realising our full potential. Bringing this into our lives means we learn to move more freely, with greater ease, flexibility and grace.

It has been said that the method can permanently improve our posture, balance and coordination, to help people in pain have a more comfortable life.

For more details take a look at the UK Feldenkrais website - http://www.feldenkrais.co.uk/

CHAPTER EIGHTEEN:
FLOTATION THERAPY.

Flotation therapy is good for back aches, pain, strains, sprains, especially those related to arthritis, traumatic injury and osteoarthritis.

The flotation tank enables you to be suspended from the effects of gravity, in a safe, warm, quiet and peaceful place, which promotes deep levels of relaxation helping ease pain, and also healing the body from the inside out.

The pressure is relieved from all your joints putting your body into a state of relaxation and kicking in your endorphins. They say one hour in the tank is the same as four hours of restful sleep which is something people in chronic pain need.

The tank contains 10 inches of super-saturated salt solution which enables you to float effortlessly on the surface. The water is heated to skin temperature and the buoyancy created by the salt solution removes the effects of gravity on the body, giving you a feeling of floating.

For years, flotation tanks were just used by researchers, but in 1983 floating increased in popularity as more was known about its effects.

Blood pressure is known to rise when you are in pain and apparently the treatment has been proven to decrease your blood pressure and your heart rate, which allows the blood to circulate in your body more efficiently.

Today you can find flotation tanks in health spas, health farms, hospitals and fitness centres.

The Flotation Tank Association is a professional organisation where you will find everything you want to know about floating and help you find your nearest FTA accredited float centre - http://flotationtankassociation.net/

CHAPTER NINETEEN:
FLOWER THERAPY.

Seasonal changes can affect people in different ways, with some feeling quite blue and low.

However the latest 'Happy Hit' is available in the form of flowers.

Flower therapy expert Clare G. Harvey suggests adding a flower essence for uplift.

'Positivity by Essence of Australia' has an exotic mix of blooms that can create a positive feeling about you. Look on this website for more details - www.flowersense.co.uk

Flower Sense has been created to serve the growing natural health community, and is committed to increasing the awareness of the remarkable healing properties of flower remedies.

The Book *'Bach Flower Remedy, The Complete Approach'*, by Mechthild Scheffer, is the most comprehensive book on Bach Flower Remedies. As well as describing the 38 remedies, it goes into the spiritual and psychological application of the therapy so that both patients and practitioners can gain deeper insight into the underlying concepts.

CHAPTER TWENTY:
GROUP THERAPY.

You read something new everyday on treatments for back pain, but now they are saying that group treatment can help pain sufferers.

A trial published in the Lancet, revealed that after only six sessions of group therapy, it showed patients still found improvements a year later.

All patients who took part in the study were given advice about remaining active, avoiding bed rest and taking pain medication, and felt more positive about being able to deal with their pain and less fearful about their situation.

The study, led by Professor Sarah Lamb at the University of Warwick, found:

"Compared with advice alone, advice plus cognitive behavioural intervention was associated with significant benefits in nearly all outcomes. This trial shows that a bespoke cognitive behavioural intervention package, Best, is effective in managing sub acute and chronic low-back pain in primary care."

The treatment also compared favourably with other ways of combating back pain, such as acupuncture and teaching correct posture.

Dr Laxmaiah Manchikanti, from the Pain Management Centre of Paducah, in Kentucky in the US, said the study *"showed rather impressive results"*.

The book *'The Theory and Practice of Group Psychotherapy'* by Irvin Yalom and Molyn Leszcz is a great book to help you understand what is behind group therapy. It presents the most recent developments in the field, drawing on nearly a decade of new research as well as the writers' clinical wisdom and expertise.

The charity MIND also have lots of details on group therapy treatments at - http://www.mind.org.uk/information-support/drugs-and-treatments/talking-treatments/#.VC8LQvldW8A

CHAPTER TWENTY ONE:
HEALING THERAPY.

'Healing' has become a popular means of alternative treatment. The scientific theory behind this is that patient's brainwaves are stimulated during the treatment, which can then help the healing process to start.

Some healers believe 'they' have been given some sort of power to help speed up the body's natural process of healing.

They say it is completely safe for people of any age or state of health. It is used for many conditions, in particular for stress and for muscoskeletal disorders and chronic illnesses. It doesn't always work but the patient usually finds that their ability to cope with their problems improves.

Many healers only require one session but usually a number of sessions are required.

The UK Confederation of Healing Organisations - website http://www.the-cho.org.uk - has everything you will want, to know about the art of healing, and one of it's aims is to ensure that the long established practice of healing becomes increasingly accepted by mainstream medicine across the UK.

My book choice on this type of healing is *Body Awareness as Healing Therapy: The Case of Nora*', by Moshe Feldenkrais. It is a classic study of a woman who has suffered a severe stroke and lost her neuromuscular coordination, including the ability to read and write.

CHAPTER TWENTY TWO:
HELLERWORK THERAPY.

Hellerwork Therapy is a movement retraining process, which focuses on the integration of the body, mind and spirit.

It's an off-shoot of rolling, craniosacral therapy and myofascial release.

It's a powerful system of somatic education and structural bodywork, and is a deep tissue bodywork combined with movement. It restores your natural balance, working from the inside by the systemic release of connective tissue.

More details are available from - www.hellerworkuk.co.uk

CHAPTER TWENTY THREE:
HOMEOPATHY.

I think it's a shame that some people talk about homoeopathy as though it was money down the drain as I'm sure most of the ones questioning it have not even tried it yet.

An article in The Mail on Sunday said that celebrity actress Nadia Sawalha's eczema drove her to 'tie her hands to the bedstead' in an attempt to stop her scratching it, then found that a controversial homoeopathy treatment cleared it up.

A homoeopathic consultant looks at the whole person to choose remedies that are decided on the basis of all aspects and symptoms the patient has.

It can help with many acute illnesses, like earache, fever, flu, tonsillitis, IBS, migraines, anxiety, depression and more. It is stated that remedies are non-addictive and they have no dangerous side effects, and are safe for the elderly, young and during pregnancies.

Nadia believed the homoeopathic cream, 'mezerum', a Eurasian shrub extract, traditionally used to heal skin complaints, was what she could only describe as 'biblical', as over 48 hours, she watched as her skin renewed itself.

There are however, still lots of sceptics, with a Professor in Edinburgh, and Pharmacists questioning that there is no evidence or scientific basis to suggest homoeopathy is an effective treatment for eczema. I guess Nadine thinks differently...

Homoeopathy is a form of alternative medicine founded by a German physician Samuel Hahnemann, himself an orthodox Doctor (MD), in 1796.

The name is derived from two Greek words that mean "like disease", basically "like cures like".

He established the law of 'similar similibus curentur' – the law of similitude – (disorders can be cured with substances which behave in a similar way). When a poison is causing certain symptoms, the same poison, but very highly-diluted, can be used to cure these symptoms.

Samuel Hahnemann was disliked by pharmacists at that time, who were the traditional suppliers of medicines to doctors, because he only needed one ingredient at a time, whereas pharmacists needed hundreds of ingredients.

He was then banned from working in different regions so he had to move his family from village to village to escape legal threats and injunctions from the medical establishment.

Homoeopathy is the third most popular method of healing in India, after conventional medicine and Ayurveda. Nine million people use it in Brazil and in some developing countries like India, Mexico and Cuba, where homoeopathy is integrated into the system of healthcare. In countries such as India, Mexico, Pakistan and South Africa, homoeopathy is on an equal level with conventional medicine, and it is also recognised in countries like Bangladesh, Singapore, Dubai, and Malaysia etc. It is also recognised in Germany, Switzerland and Canada and in countries such as Australia and New Zealand, where it's developing into a complete healthcare profession and is receiving government recognition.

The theory is actually quite simple, as they just take all the patient's symptoms, and then find a matching remedy, i.e., something that could cause similar symptoms in a healthy person.

A qualified and experienced homoeopath can sometimes cure serious chronic diseases when traditional medicine can do nothing further, and when used in the right way.

The treatments are made from the elements found in nature, i.e., mineral, animal and plant extracts, which are the bases of the remedies which are then diluted to avoid side-effects. By knowing the toxic effects of herb, mineral or animal fluid, a homoeopath can then turn it into a homoeopathic remedy which will then have the direct opposite effect and with no side effects or reactions.

Apparently, according to an article in Woman & Home, 'a whole cast list of celebs, and the Queen' use Homoeopathy for treating different conditions.

Homoeopathy is a 200 year-old holistic healing method, where a substance that causes symptoms when it's taken in large doses, can, when used in highly-diluted amounts, treat those same symptoms. You can buy remedies over the counter, but for a serious condition it's best if you visit a Homoeopath to discuss your needs. You usually need at least one or two different types of homoeopathic medicine to help with your problems, but it's usually not too expensive and has no known side-effects.

Some Homoeopathic websites to check out are 'The Faculty of Homoeopathy', - www.britishhomeopathic.org - and 'The Society of Homoeopaths', - www.homeopathy-soh.org

You can buy your remedies at 'Ainsworths' - www.ainsworths.com - who reputedly hold royal warrants from the Queen and Prince Charles for their homoeopathic remedies.

'The Organic Pharmacy' - www.theorganicpharmacy.com - which is modern and helpful. 'Helios Homepage' - www.helios.co.uk - which has great first-aid kits and soothing creams.

My choice of book is 'The Complete Homoeopathy Handbook' by Miranda Castro, a guide to everyday health healthcare, and an absolutely brilliant complete book on Homoeopathy.

CHAPTER TWENTY FOUR:
HYPNOTHERAPY.

In England, around 1843, the surgeon, James Braid, revisited the phenomenon of Mesmerism and renamed it hypnosis, after the Greek God of sleep, Hypnos. He was the first person to attribute the phenomenon to psychological rather than physical variables. His findings renewed interest in the subject, especially in France, where hypnosis gained popularity again as a form of pain reduction during surgery. Eventually, Braid's technique was found to be unsatisfactory, and hypnosis drifted out of favour again.

So, just what is hypnosis? Hypnotherapists say it's a way to focus one's imagination and attention to help alleviate physical and emotional problems. Brain-imaging has shown that some hypnotic suggestions reduce activity in brain areas associated with emotional responses to pain, while other suggestions reduce activity in an area of the brain more directly involved with the physical sensation of pain.

Most hypnotherapists have patients stare at a fixed object, sometimes just a coloured thumb tack stuck in a wall. The hypnotherapist then describes relaxing images, such as a walk along a beach, and asks the patient to focus on those images. Next, he uses imagery and suggestions to block out or transform pain, such as, *"Lock away the pain in the box in the basement of an abandoned house."*

While hypnosis typically helps relieve pain in four to 10 sessions, some people benefit faster and others not at all. Practitioners usually teach ways to continue therapy at home, and as long as the techniques are followed, people may not have to return for further sessions.

Hypnosis is thought to work by altering our state of consciousness in such a way that the analytical left-hand side of the brain is turned off, while the non-analytical right-hand side is made more alert. The conscious control of the mind is inhibited, and the subconscious mind awoken. Since the subconscious mind is a deeper-seated, more instinctive force than the conscious mind, this is the part which has to change for the patient's behaviour and physical state to alter. There are lots of books on this type of therapy but Paul McKenna's books seem to stay at the top of the Amazon list.

My own GP performed hypnosis on me after I kept having flash backs from a very unpleasant life-threatening episode. The episode involved a treatment I underwent in a hospital but it left me terrified of going in any hospital and every time I went to sleep the flash backs came.The treatment worked for me in this instance and yet not for pain relief.

To find a qualified hypnotherapist, ask your doctor for a referral. Or to find a registered hypnotherapist head to the UK Association website - http://www.thehypnotherapyassociation.co.uk/

CHAPTER TWENTY FIVE:
HYDROTHERAPY.

Research has shown that if you suffer from osteoarthritis pain in the knee or hip, then aerobic and stretching exercises in warm water can help to relieve it.

There are three categories of exercises called hydrotherapy: hot water, cold water, and alternating hot and cold water.

Hot water is known for stimulating the immune system and is also good with increasing your circulation. Cold water constricts blood vessels and is effective in reducing inflammation. Using both hot and cold has been found to improve circulation.

It was found that water heated to between 32 degrees C to 36 degrees C slightly reduces osteoarthritis pain over three months.

They say that hydrotherapy changes lives and has been proven to be a highly-effective form of natural therapy which works by stimulating the endorphins, which in turn helps you to control pain and alleviate tension.

The hydro bath works by releasing millions of large bubbles, which relax your muscular tension and helps reduce swollen joints, giving you increased mobility and more importantly lessens your pain. It is available on the NHS and a good website to find out more about it is the Hydrotherapy UK Association - http://www.hydrotherapy.org.uk/

CHAPTER TWENTY SIX:
HANNA SOMATIC EDUCATION THERAPY.

Hanna Somatic Education (aka HSE) teaches you how to release muscles that have involuntarily contracted.

There are only a few Somatic therapists in the UK and one is Jonathan Hunt, a former Premiership footballer who had to retire in 2003 due to back pain.

When manipulative therapies failed to help him, he tried the Hanna Somatic programme and was so impressed that he trained as a therapist himself.

Some of the suggested exercises for backache are:

Lie on your back, arms resting by your side, knees bent, and feet hip-width apart tucked up near your bottom.

As you breathe in, arch your lower back by pressing your tail bone down, then very slowly flatten your back into the floor as you exhale, to relax.

Rest, and then repeat slowly and gently ten to 15 times. When you finish, straighten and stretch your legs.

Don't attempt any of these until you have checked with your GP first and don't overdo them as they should be comfortable.

Jonathan's details are - www.somaticliving.com

CHAPTER TWENTY SEVEN:
INFRA-RED LIGHT THERAPY.

Infra-red Light Therapy for pain is being called 'The best kept secret for pain relief'.

Natural and safe, infra-red therapy is recommended for the relief of muscular pain, sore muscles, arthritis, bursitis, backache, tennis elbow, joint pain and related pains.

All you do is aim the light to the painful area, then the deep penetrating infra-red energy will be felt as gentle warmth in the treated area. Taut muscles will then loosen up to give much needed relief.

Its 200w infra-red warmth is very comfortable and penetrates deep into the skin, improving blood circulation, and this begins the healing process as pain is relieved.

Philips makes a 200w infra-red light for £39.99, which states:

'Philips Infra care gives effective pain relief for muscles and joints'.

Another plus point of course is that there are no side-effects, but just like anything else you might try, speak with your GP before buying one of these units.

I cannot find any books on this subject but a great website that explains it all is - 'Time to Heal - https://sites.google.com/a/timetoheal.co.za/www/professional-massage/infrared-light-therapy

CHAPTER TWENTY EIGHT:
JOURNAL THERAPY.

Some people say that keeping a journal is the cheapest kind of therapy you can have. All you need is some paper or a notebook and something to write with. Personally, I use a pencil as I find this easier to write with than a pen.

Things you could write about are:

- Write it daily or weekly and write how your day went and what the next few days hold for you.
- List the best things that have happened that week/day/month or year in your life.
- Describe the worst thing that has ever happened to you.
- Write your own prayer.
- Describe a special moment.
- Write your own mantra.
- Write a dialogue with another person, or describe an event, a part of your body, or a famous person.
- Make a list of your activities, your stresses, your fears, your hopes. What makes you sad/happy and/or your favourite people.
- Write what you have enjoyed watching on the television.
- Write about the weather.

Keeping it as something that you do 'when you feel like it', as opposed to 'must be written' will, in the end, make it a much nicer experience. It's also nice to look back over and read a few years on.

My book of choice on this (and there are many) is 'The Write Therapy: How Keeping A Journal Can Make You Happier, Healthier and More Productive', by Lyn Alderson.

CHAPTER TWENTY NINE:
KINESIOLOGY THERAPY.

Kinesiology is a treatment which concentrates on getting your muscles to function correctly. It is believed that each muscle is connected to a specific part of your body.

The word 'Kinesiology' is derived from the Greek word 'kinesis', which means 'motion'. The treatment originated in 1964 and was developed by an American chiropractor called George Goodheart. He found that when he was treating patients for severe pain in the leg, that by massaging particular muscles the pain seemed to ease. However this did not seem to work on all muscles.

An osteopath in the 1900's, Dr. Chapman, pointed out that there were certain 'pressure points' in the body which were connected to your muscles, and if these were massaged correctly the lymph would be able to flow freely throughout the body.

In the 1930's, it was also claimed that there were similar pressure points which were on the skull which, by putting a light pressure on them, the flow of blood to their related organs would be assisted.

A Kinesiologist will examine a patient and try to discover whether they are lacking in energy as well as any other problems which could relate to their symptoms. If they find blockages then they can treat the disorder by stimulating the flow of lymph and blood by massaging the pressure points.

Nowadays there are a number of therapies (acupuncture, osteopathy, Myofascial release massage, etc.,) that use pressure points to ease pain in the muscles.

After treatment by massage of the pressure points, the patient would experience some tenderness for a couple of days as the toxins in the tissue dissipate gradually. However, there should be an overall feeling of an improvement in your health and in particular the areas that were treated.

http://www.therapyworks.com.au/a/42.html

CHAPTER THIRTY:
KNITTING THERAPY.

Knitting has become so popular that Simple Knitting weekends are available in Cornwall.

Knitting has proved a perfect way to switch off and relax, and even better than meditation which some people find hard to practice.

The courses are run by knitting expert, Erika Knight, at the Bethruthn Steps Hotel in Pawgan Porth.

Knitting groups are also popping up all over the country, where you can meet up with fellow knitters and catch up on all the gossip while knitting.

They say that knitting has many health benefits including reducing stress and anxiety, and alleviating depression and some pain.

A physiotherapist (Betsan Corkhill) is so convinced of it that she has set up a knitting group in the Chronic Pain Unit at the Royal United Hospital in Bath and founded www.stitchlinks.com which aims to provide support and friendship through knitting and stitching worldwide.

Experts feel that there's a neurochemical effect on the brain which undoubtedly changes brain chemistry for the better, possibly by decreasing stress hormones and increasing feel-good serotonin and dopamine, while knitting.

CHAPTER THIRTY ONE:
KRIOTHERAPY.

Kriotherapy is the latest feel-good therapy which has apparently been known to heal muscular injuries, chronic aches and pains, help alleviate arthritis, boost circulation, the immune system, and help with fatigue, insomnia and the central nervous system.

It involves spending two to three minutes at a temperature between -60 degrees C and -135 degrees C, depending on your size and fitness level. It is stated that it is not suitable for people who suffer from claustrophobia and no-one should undertake it until a full medical history has been taken.

You are put in front of a fan to dry out your body thoroughly then put into a cabinet where the dry ice begins to seep in while you acclimatise to the -60 degrees C, then another door opens where you are in a -135 degrees C atmosphere. After three minutes you are put through your paces to help the released blood (which is sent out to protect vital organs in freezing temperatures) surge through your body, with ten minutes on the treadmill, an exercise bike and exercises.

The fact that you are cold, and then warm, apparently makes the blood swirl into action to help heal. The kriotherapy room at Champneys health resort near Tring, Hertfordshire, is kept at a staggering minus 130 degrees C - brrrrrrrr!

I'm not sure if I'd fancy this and wonder if ice packs, followed by warm packs, would hit the spot just the same?

CHAPTER THIRTY TWO:
LOW LEVEL LASER THERAPY.

Low level laser therapy is a red or near infra-red light, applied from a low power laser specifically for therapeutic usage, where the light penetrates deep into the tissues.

Apart from it being used for back pain, it is also employed to treat musculo-skeletal injuries and disorders, as well as Fibromyalgia.

A low-level laser differs in that it operates at very low levels of power and unlike high-power lasers it does not heat or damage human tissue.

It can help back pain by reducing pain and inflammation. You would probably need several treatments before you notice much pain relief and combined with exercise can be more beneficial than exercise alone. They call it the cutting edge of non-surgical pain relief and tissue repair.

Laser therapy uses light waves to stimulate healing in soft tissues. It has a similar effect to ultrasound. It is a low level cold laser and is pain free; it works from the infra-red spectrum which penetrates up to 3cm into the muscles tendons and ligaments of the body.

The laser light then stimulates the cell body within muscles, tendons or ligaments causing them to oxidise and increase healing at twice the normal rate.

It can improve healing, pain reduction, increase circulation and decrease swellings. It is not available on the NHS, but there are a number of clinics throughout the UK which perform this type of pain relief.

Some sites to look at - www.birminghamchiropracticclinic.co.uk and www.citybackpainclinic.co.uk

CHAPTER THIRTY THREE:
LIGHT THERAPY.

Light therapy is a treatment mainly used to treat SAD (Seasonal Affective Disorder) and depression. But it is now recommended for a number of other complaints including chronic pain and chronic fatigue.

Exposure to the light is thought to alter your Circadian Rhythms and suppress your body's natural release of melatonin which is a hormone that helps regulate sleep.

Based on NASA 'research on healing' using LED lights, it is safe, effective, affordable, soothing, relieves stiffness, chronic pain and is a safe alternative to drugs.

The light can help to increase circulation which helps to alleviate joint stiffness as well as reduce some of the swelling that may be causing your pain.

It uses specific wavelengths of light or even daylight, to help relieve pain.

Other benefits include experiencing pleasant warm and tingling sensations, a stimulation of collagen production and an increase in energy.

Philips manufactures a few types of infra-red therapy light boxes - the infra care HP3621 or the HP3631, which are quite reasonable in price.

CHAPTER THIRTY FOUR:
MEDITATION THERAPY.

Many people are turning to meditation as an effective way to relax and bring inner peace.

It can also help with stress, improve your general health and help you to think clearly. It's something you can do wherever you are, by focusing on something else around you instead of your thoughts, worries and obsessions. You can meditate just by focusing on something; anything will do if you are out. But most people still meditate on breathing, a single repeated word, a flower or a mental image. Meditation is much more than just a way of relaxing, it also clears our minds and makes us more alert. If you meditate for a few minutes each day, the results can be deep and long-lasting. There are many places you can learn to meditate; it could be a candle-lit room, with incense and dreamy music, lying on the floor after a yoga class or at an evening's class at your local school or leisure centre.

In your first meditation, people may feel sleepy as they let themselves relax and their adrenalin levels drop. They will go to classes after a hard day's work, and need to rest. Meditation is not about going to sleep. It's about learning to relax and focus your mind. The benefits of meditation ripple through everything we do - being relaxed and aware is the mental equivalent of being fit and healthy. Some of the main reasons people meditate are for relaxation, health, inner peace and harmony, concentration to improve sporting and theatrical performance, inspiration and creativity, quality of life, self-understanding and therapy and spiritual awakening - the list goes on.

'Mindfulness Meditation' is a very simple way to meditate. All you do is focus on your breathing, observe your thoughts and bring your attention into the present moment. Meditation is thought to date back to the fifth and sixth century BC. Stories were written in ancient Hindu about it, and are featured in most religions. Ed Halliwell, author of 'The Mindful Manifesto,' says that 'it can help you experience the moment and not be drawn into habitual emotional responses'. Halliwell goes on to say that 'research on human brains during a meditation state has revealed a shift in activity from the right side of the pre-frontal cortex, which is linked with depression, over to the left, which is connected with emotional reassurance and happiness'.

Research has actually shown meditation can ease depression, lower the risk of cardiovascular disease, boost immunity and healing, and lower blood pressure. Mindfulness meditation is now an NHS approved treatment. You can find a course or practise it on your own.

For more details go to the website www.themindfulmanifesto.com.

CHAPTER THIRTY FIVE:
MIND-BODY THERAPY.

Reuters Health has found that a form of 'mind-body' therapy, which focuses on the role of emotions in physical pain, may offer some relief to people who suffer from Fibromyalgia, a small recent study suggests.

Even though many people suffer from Fibromyalgia, the actual cause is unknown. There are no physical signs, such as inflammation and tissue damage in the painful area, although some researchers believe the disorder involves problems with how the brain processes pain signals.

Standard treatments include painkillers, antidepressants, cognitive-behavioural therapy and exercise therapy. Part of that, according to the researchers on the new study, may be because standard treatments do not specifically address the role psychological stress and emotions can play in triggering people's pain.

That is not to say that the pain people with Fibromyalgia feel is "all in their head," stressed Dr. Howard Schubiner, of St. John Health/Providence Hospital and Medical Centres in Southfield, Michigan.

"The pain is very real," Schubiner said in an interview. But, he explained, pain and emotions are *"connected in the brain,"* and emotional factors may act to trigger *"learned nerve pathways"* that give rise to pain.

For the new study, published in the Journal of General Internal Medicine, Schubiner and his colleagues tested the effects of affective self-awareness, a technique Schubiner developed and uses in treating certain chronic pain conditions, including Fibromyalgia.

They randomly assigned 45 women with the condition to either undergo the therapy or go on a waiting-list for treatment, serving as a control group. Women in the treatment group each had a one-on-one consultation, and then attended three group meetings to learn the affective self-awareness techniques so that they could carry them out on their own.

The therapy involves an educational component, where patients learn about the emotion-pain connection. They learn specific techniques, including mindfulness meditation and "expressive" writing, for recognising and dealing with the emotions that may be contributing to their pain.

Patients are also encouraged to get back to any exercise or other activities that they have been avoiding due to pain.

Schubiner's team found that six months later, 46 percent of the treatment group had at least a 30% reduction in their pain ratings, compared with scores at the outset. 21 percent had a 50% or greater reduction.

None of the women in the control group had a comparable improvement.

The study is only the first clinical trial to test affective self-awareness for Fibromyalgia, and it had a number of limitations, including its small size.

In addition, the control group received no active therapy to serve as a comparison. That is important because it is possible for patients to benefit from simply receiving attention from a healthcare provider, or being part of small-group sessions with other people suffering from the same condition, for example.

Schubiner also acknowledged that this general "model" for understanding and addressing Fibromyalgia pain is controversial.

He said that he and his colleagues have applied for funding to conduct a larger clinical trial comparing affective self-awareness with standard cognitive-behavioural therapy.

Affective self-awareness and cognitive-behavioural therapy have similarities, according to Schubiner. Both, for example, try to show patients that they have the power to improve their own health.

A key difference, Schubiner said, is that affective self-awareness asks people to "directly engage" the emotions that may be helping to drive their symptoms.

Another difference is that, right now, only a small number of healthcare providers practice affective self-awareness, according to Schubiner.

Some components of the technique, such as teachings in mindfulness meditation, are more widely available. But whether those practices in isolation would help 'Fibromyalgia patients' pain is not clear.

CHAPTER THIRTY SIX:
MOIST HEAT THERAPY.

Moist heat is nothing like all other heat appliances, like pads and water bottles. Moist heat is from a shower, whirlpool, warm swimming pool, steam room or bath.

Some Doctors apparently say that using moist heat treatments twice a day will be more productive in reducing pain than other types of heat methods.

The goal is for the heat to penetrate deep into your muscles, which can then reduce stiffness, relax your muscles and increase circulation.

There is a difference between moist heat therapy and dry heat therapy. Using a heating pad is applying dry heat. Using moisture wraps, hot baths, showers, whirlpool and steamed towels are what constitute moist therapy.

The difference between the two is that the dry heat can dehydrate your skin as the heat draws out the moisture, whereas the moist heat does not dry out your skin. Instead, it penetrates into the joints, soft tissues and muscles.

CHAPTER THIRTY SEVEN:
MUSIC THERAPY.

Music therapy has also been found to reduce the disability, anxiety, and depression associated with chronic pain.

A study carried out in Ohio suggests that listening to music may help to alleviate pain.

Patients who listened to music on headsets for an hour every day for a week reported that their pain had reduced by between 12% and 21%. They were also less depressed and felt they had more control over their pain.

A good site for some calming music to buy is - www.calmtime.com

CHAPTER THIRTY EIGHT:
MYOFASCIAL RELEASE THERAPY.

I started with a new type of pain relief called 'Myofascial release', which my pain consultant thought I would benefit from, as he felt a lot of my pain is 'Myofascial pain'.

They call it a form of soft tissue therapy intended for pain relief, increasing your range of motion and balancing the body.

There are now lots of articles online, raving about pain relief using this technique, and many more on how you can treat yourself.

In America, sufferers are doing 'self-myofascial release (foam rolling)' using a lacrosse ball and foam to roll out trigger points.

They say, *'it can help reduce muscle soreness, increase mobility, and prevent problems created by tightness and poor tissue quality like plantar fascists, sciatica, and more."*

It is a scientific fact that all muscles and their fibrous coating and connective tissue that joins muscles to bones, the fascia, are a source of pain if the functionality is changed by an accident or normal wear and tear/degeneration.

Muscles may develop Myofascial 'tender spots' or 'Trigger Points'. These Trigger Points are not only painful where they are found, but may also send pain away from that spot, to what is called Referred pain. All the body's 600 plus muscles have an area in the muscle that is tender to pressure.

There are YouTube videos, showing you how to lie on your foam roller to release your tight spine. This technique is gaining popularity every day and has become very popular among athletes and serious fitness enthusiasts.

I've had a number of treatments and there is no question that it does release the taut muscles which then release pain, but the relief did not last long enough for me. I wasn't expecting miracles to happen but I was hoping for longer pain relief.

The National Association of Myofascial Trigger Point Therapists is a good place to start to find a qualified therapist - http://www.myofascialtherapy.org/ - and another good book on the subject is *'Myofascial Release: Your Guide to Myofascial Release with a Tennis Ball'* by Merl Buchreich.

CHAPTER THIRTY NINE:
MICKEL THERAPY.

Mickel Therapy was developed in the UK by medical doctor, Dr. David Mickel, for the treatment of Chronic Fatigue Syndrome, ME, Fibromyalgia, MS, anxiety, depression, IBS and some types of back pain.

Mickel Therapy is a one-to-one talking session between two people, the therapist and yourself. It involves no medication, dietary change, supplements or psychotherapy of any sort.

Treatments are a series of one hour sessions, during which you will learn why your symptoms are there and, crucially, how to work with them to regain your health.

The treatment can also be administered by email, telephone/webcam or a combination of both.

Mickel Therapy believes that a part of the brain (Hypothalamus) which is responsible for keeping your systems in balance, is working too fast, and that's why people suffering feel overwhelming tiredness, as well as a number of other symptoms.

It is the role of the therapist to help you to see why you have symptoms and gives you easy to follow tools that help prove for yourself how you can in fact rid yourself of the symptoms. The therapy works in between your sessions with the therapist, with your own participation.

The actual notion of a talking therapy to help you free you of a hugely debilitating physical condition can sound a bit far-fetched, but the reported success rate apparently speaks for itself.

On the main website it states that 'to date, over 2000 people have successfully applied the tools and techniques of Mickel Therapy for CFS, ME, Fibromyalgia and other conditions'.

A list of Mickel Therapy UK Practicioners is available from this website - http://www.mickeltherapy.com/practitioners/

CHAPTER FORTY:
MAGNET THERAPY.

The Chinese use magnets, as well as acupuncture, and say the difference is just that needles work faster, but that magnets applied correctly are just as effective for some complaints. They also think that the magnets are thought to stimulate the body's 'chi' to promote healing.

Apparently, Cleopatra is said to have worn a polished lodestone on her 3rd eye to maintain her beauty!

Although magnets became popular in the 19th and 20th centuries, the medical profession was against the use of them, but since then, magnets and magnetic products have become more and more popular with an increase in scientific studies showing the effectiveness of them.

At the moment the jury is still out as to whether the use of magnets for health problems is truly beneficial or just provides a placebo effect. But, unless people continually try out these different types of therapies for pain, we cannot get scientific research and feedback produced.

Some good websites to browse through with magnets for sale are - www.therionmagnetics.com, - www.synergyforlife.com , - www.lifes2good.com and a great book on the subject is 'Magnet Therapy: Second Edition', by William H Philpott and Dwight K Kalita.

CHAPTER FORTY ONE:
MASSAGE THERAPY.

Body massage is a great way to keep your mind and body conditioned for your day to day activities at work, school and at home.

Massage therapy is beneficial for you physically, emotionally, and psychologically. Aside from the fact that it relaxes our muscles and relieves us of pain and stress, the constant skin-to-skin contact has been known to have positive effects on self-esteem and self-image.

For example, a Swedish massage, called Effleurage, promotes relaxation and releases muscle tension through smooth, gliding strokes,.

Aromatherapy body massage, on the other hand, uses essential oils to reinforce the relaxing effect of a massage. These essential oils can either energise, reduce stress or balance hormone levels. This type of body massage is suitable for soothing stress-related ailments.

There are also certain body massages that are designed to help heal injured muscles and connective tissues. The deep tissue massage is one particular technique that caters to such a need. A deep tissue massage is a technique that focuses on deeper muscles and connective tissues. Sustained muscle injuries can heal faster with properly applied pressure and strokes from a deep tissue massage.

Research has shown that the strokes employed in sports massage reduce lactic acid that causes muscle spasms and cramps during physical activities. Athletes often ask their massage therapists to be there before and during competitions, because it helps them warm up for the upcoming activity. When muscles are properly warmed-up, they are also more likely to perform better. The key to a good sports massage is to focus on the muscle to be used. For instance, arms, back, and legs are targeted for boxing matches, while legs and feet muscles are the focus for ice skaters and hockey players.

If you can't get to a therapist then you could try massaging with a tennis ball. Always knead your limbs in the direction of your heart. For general aches, pains and tiredness simply roll your feet over the tennis ball in order to stimulate acupoints that will help your whole body to relax. To relieve pressure on your spine, tilt your feet to work the instep.

A good book to read on different types of massage is called 'The Book of Massage: The Complete Step By Step Guide to Eastern and Western Techniques', by Lucinda Lidell.

If you have never before had a back massage, you must put it down on your to do list. You can usually find lots of vouchers online or via their associations website - http://www.nammt.co.uk/

CHAPTER FORTY TWO:
OCCUPATIONAL THERAPY.

Occupational therapy is given to you by a therapist who is someone who can check your posture at work and at home.

Bad posture and poor work related positions can play havoc with your back and neck and, over time it can also aggravate other health problems.

The Occupational therapist can check your work-related positions and posture and suggest ways to help alleviate your pain at work or your work at home.

They can also provide advice, look at ways an everyday task can be done differently; recommend alterations or changes at home; refer you to other services to help you and help you address work-related issues.

Occupational therapists have specialist knowledge and can advise you on disability equipment, housing adaptations and adaptations to the workplace.

They are available through the NHS and your GP can put you in contact with your nearest therapist.

CHAPTER FORTY THREE:
OSTEOPATHY.

Osteopathy is an alternative medical technique that uses manipulation and massage to help distressed muscles and joints, to help them work smoothly.

Treatment can improve many parts of the body by restoring normal movement in areas that have become dysfunctional. This can then allow the tissue to nourish, replenish and repair in a more natural way.

The treatment first began in 1892 when a Dr. Andrew Taylor Still (1828-1917), an American farmer, inventor and doctor, opened the first school of osteopathic medicine in the USA. He looked for alternatives to medical treatments in his day which he felt were ineffective as well as harmful.

His new philosophy of medicine was based on the teachings of Hippocrates. The therapy aims to pinpoint and treat any problems that are of a mechanical nature. Our body's frame consists of the skeleton, muscles, joints and ligaments and all movements or activities such as running, swimming, eating, speaking and walking depend on it.

When you first see an Osteopath, he or she will need to know the complete history of any problems you have, how they first occurred and what eases or aggravates matters, so a diary kept over a week or more before your visit would be a great help.

Osteopathy is a way of detecting, treating and preventing health problems by moving, stretching and massaging a person's muscles and joints. It is based on the principle that the well-being of an individual depends on their bones, muscles, ligaments and connective tissue functioning smoothly together.

Ostepaths believe their treatments allow the body to heal itself. You should always check that the therapist is fully qualified and can find therapists on the Osteopath Association website - http://www.osteopathy.org/

CHAPTER FORTY FOUR:
PHYSICAL THERAPY.

Physical Therapy can be administered in three different ways to relieve back pain.

The three treatments are traction, massage, and direct applications of heat and/or cold.

Traction uses mechanical apparatus to stretch the back muscles and ligaments in order to relieve the pressure on spinal nerves and inter-vertebral discs.

Back in the 1970's traction was commonly used as the first port of call for disc problems. I was on traction for a week for my first prolapsed disc, which seemed to help it a little but left me with some numbness in my lower left limb.

I was also put on neck traction for a disc problem in my cervical area which was not successful and actually resulted in emergency surgery. So, I'm not really an advocate of this type of treatment for back pain. Nowadays it's used less for in-patient treatment, but is still used quite frequently in physiotherapy departments.

CHAPTER FORTY FIVE:
POLARITY THERAPY.

This therapy was devised by Dr. Randolph Stone (1890-1983), and amalgamates other healing therapies from both east and west.

Dr. Stone studied many therapies, such as yoga and acupuncture, osteopathy and chiropractic. Through his studies, he believed that a form of energy flows along certain channels in the body and that to keep good health the flow must be maintained.

In India, this therapy is referred to as 'Prama' and in China, it is called 'Chi' or 'Gi'. They believe that illness occurs when this flow of energy is blocked or is out of balance, and that once the flow of energy has been restored to normal, the ailment would disappear and not recur.

The process incorporates three levels of touch - 'very light', 'stimulating', and 'deep'. It is important to note that, if you do not wish to have touch contact, the therapist will respect your wishes. This process can be relaxing and restorative and can also allow emotional and personal issues to surface and become clearer.

For a back pain treatment, they first work to loosen tight muscles in your back to ease the pain.

The final part of the treatment concentrates on mental attitude, which is basically a way of encouraging people to have a more positive view on all aspects of their lives, through talking and counselling sessions.

For Polarity Therapy to truly work, you need to believe in it completely and be prepared to carry out your practitioner's instructions with regard to diet, exercises etc.

This type of therapy is often found with other eastern remedies that have the common themes of contemplation, exercise, touch or pressure, and diet.

More details can be found at - http://www.polarity.tk/ - which is the UK Polarity Association website.

CHAPTER FORTY SIX:
PET THERAPY.

As I'm sure most of us pet owners know, a pet can be a great comfort to you at the best of times. Now, various studies have shown some remarkable health benefits of owning an animal.

It's what is thought to be the *'wonderful, wide-ranging biochemical and physiological effects pets can have on those suffering from chronic pain and fibromyalgia'*.

Smaller dogs in particular have been of benefit to 'fibro' sufferers, who cannot get out much. Through their unconditional love, dogs can encourage you to be a little more active, feel more secure, and help your mood.

Pet therapy is used in some hospitals and care homes; just the simple act of petting a dog can have a calming effect on people and have a knock-on effect with lowering stress levels and anxiety.

'Pets as Therapy' is a national therapy founded in 1983, which provides therapeutic visits to hospitals, hospices, care homes and special needs schools.

It can be found at - http://www.petsastherapy.org/

There's a lovely article in *'The Power of Pets'* by Sally Abrahms, which is well worth reading.

CHAPTER FORTY SEVEN:
QIGONG THERAPY.

This is a form of Chinese medicine which helps increase energy, alleviate pain and ease fatigue. All of which sounds like a miracle to me!

When employing this technique, you will move into specific physical postures to help ease tension over your whole body.

It is similar to the theory of ying and yang, and that everything is related. In traditional Chinese medicine, Qi is treated as the fundamental substance of the human body, and its movements explain various life processes.

Qigong (also spelled Ch'i Kung) is a powerful system of healing and energy medicine from China.

It is the art and science of using breathing techniques, gentle movement, and meditation to cleanse, strengthen, and circulate the life energy (Qi) which I have written about earlier.

Qigong practice leads to better health and vitality and a tranquil state of mind. In the past, qigong was also called Nei Gong (inner work) and Dao Yin (guiding energy).

CHAPTER FORTY EIGHT:
REIKI THERAPY.

Reiki (pronounced Ray-key) is a complementary therapy which was named after Dr. Mikao Usui, a Japanese theologist.

Reiki is a Japanese word, meaning Universal Life Energy, an energy which is all around us. It is regarded as 'life's energy' and creates a feeling of deep relaxation.

Energy blockages are removed, allowing a free flow of life energy throughout the body. Toxins are removed from the body with other waste products leaving the system much more quickly.

Then, with the toxins removed from your body, more energy can be received and your vital processors and functions become more highly tuned.

The hands are the main instrument used in the healing by Reiki, and can be effective through clothing. It has also been useful for anyone taking drugs to help reduce some of the side effects. They say it is possible to heal acute injuries but chronic injuries can take longer to heal.

Reiki is a therapy available to anyone, and can help the receiver of the therapy to achieve a more relaxed approach to life and greater harmony.

On the UK Reiki Federation website - http://www.reikifed.co.uk/ - you can find all you need to know about this type of therapy as well as finding yourself a good therapist.

My book of choice on this subject, of which there are many is 'Essential Reiki: A Complete Guide to an Ancient Healing Art' by Diana Stein.

CHAPTER FORTY NINE:
RELAXATION THERAPY.

Many people think that relaxation means sitting in front of the television, or going on holiday, but in actual fact, it can be taken by doing your favourite sport.

You can relax when you are swimming, cycling, walking, doing yoga, aerobics, playing golf, and so on.

The best way to look after your body is to find ways to help you relax. Normal stress is a challenge which strengthens the body's own defences. However, abnormal stress and too much of it, can overtax us physically as well as mentally.

The NHS site says *"Having a massage is no better at beating stress than home relaxation techniques, like breathing deeply and listening to soothing music,"* reports The Daily Telegraph.

This news is based on a trial on the effectiveness of therapeutic massage in treating generalised anxiety disorder (GAD), compared to thermotherapy (a heat-based treatment) or relaxation room therapy. After 12 weeks, anxiety scores improved in all three groups. If you are getting a sudden searing pain in your back, then try 'The Jacobson Technique', also called Progressive Muscle Relaxation, which has been around for 100 years. The Jacobson technique is commonly used for pain management for all kinds of conditions.

Jacobson's relaxation technique was developed by Dr. Edmund Jacobson over half a century ago. Jacobson formulated over 200 exercises and techniques which, taken together, relax the entire body by releasing muscular tension that accumulates as a person experiences a stressful situation.

Jacobson, and those who have followed in his footsteps, claim that this technique will cure not only tight muscles and cramps, but also reduces the intensity of pain, and will relieve stress and anxiety.

Today, the 200 exercises developed by Jacobson have been reduced to between 15 and 20. In order to receive maximum benefit, it is recommended to practice this technique every day for at least 20 minutes, at the same time every day, in a quiet, comfortable place.

Jacobson founded the International Stress Management Association, which continues his work to this day. The International Stress Management Association (ISMA) produces publications and offers trainings in Jacobson's relaxation therapy at - http://www.isma.org.uk/

CHAPTER FIFTY:
REFLEXOLOGY.

Reflexology is a holistic treatment, based on the principle that there are areas and points on the feet, hands, and ears that map via the nervous system to corresponding parts of the body. When pressure is applied to these areas and points it stimulates the movement of energy along the nerve channels, and helps to restore homoeostasis (balance) in the whole body.

There are 7000-7200 nerve endings in the human foot, and each of these is a reflex point that corresponds to a body part. Reflexologists know which area of the foot corresponds to which part of the body by learning maps of the feet.

Reflexology has been practised in some form, for thousands of years. In fact, the first solid proof was found on a pictograph painted on an Egyptian tomb dated between 2500-2330 BC.

The next evidence came in the form of a book written by two physicians called Dr Adamus and Dr Atitis on zone therapy in 1582. Another picture shows the practice in China, dated 1870.

Reflexology is an excellent whole body system, and can be used both to prevent illness and to encourage the body to heal. It is particularly useful for stress and related disorders, emotional disorders, digestive problems, circulatory disorders, menstrual problems, insomnia, fatigue and most chronic and acute illnesses.

A brilliant book on Reflexology is 'The Reflexology Bible: The Definitive Guide to Reflexology', by Louise Keet.

I have regular reflexology treatments and find that it helps with my sleep, which in turn helps with my pain. The UK Association of Reflexology is another great site to find out all about this type of treatment and where to find a therapist.

Visit - http://www.britreflex.co.uk/

CHAPTER FIFTY ONE:
SHOE THERAPY.

I bet you never thought you would see a therapy for shoes! Sorry, but I couldn't resist putting this in the book. For ladies only, I'm afraid!

'Shoetherapy' sell supportive ballet pumps, which are great for back pain sufferers who cannot wear heels. Their website says 'banish back pain and embrace fashion.'

The special sole relieves back and joint pain and can improve circulation to your legs. They were developed ten years ago by a French orthopaedic doctor, especially for nurses on their feet all day.

Because they are sturdier than a traditional pump, it means that you don't feel every lump and bump on the pavement.

They say that they have been scientifically tested and clinical trials prove a reduction of up to 75% of back and joint pains experienced by women.

The patented sole is also designed to minimise strain on the calf muscles and improve poor circulation, which in turn helps prevent the appearance of varicose veins and cellulite.

To find out more or to buy a pair, head to their website at - http://www.shoetherapy.com/

CHAPTER FIFTY TWO:
TAI CHI.

According to a recent article in 'Arthritis Today', Tai Chi can be effective in managing chronic low back pain.

The study from Australia showed that people experienced a 25% reduction in their pain intensity, when they completed the Tai Chi programme.

Apparently, this is the first randomised, controlled trial to see the effects of the ancient mind/body exercise on the reduction of lower back pain.

Apart from it promoting the flow of Qi energy, Tai Chi also helps increase flexibility, suppleness and exercises the muscles. The smooth, gentle movements help to relax you and keep your mind calm and focused.

To put it into perspective, 23% reported an improvement with their pain, and 32% reported an improvement with their disability, after completing a Tai Chi course. However, scientists believe that the 'positive' results only last for as long as the patient takes part in the Tai Chi exercises.

Tai Chi is thought of as a moving form of yoga and meditation combined. It is accessible to all ages and physical abilities and can be practised on many levels, from a simple 'meditative' exercise to a martial art.

This is a new therapy to me, so I cannot really comment, but I have been to two classes and came home and had the best night's sleep I have had in years. The best part is that you don't even work up a sweat, even though you seem to be moving every muscle in your body. I found the breathing exercises extremely good.

Finding the right book on this subject is hard, as there are so many out there, and after chatting to my teacher, I think the best way to look at this type of therapy would be by going to YouTube and checking out some of the videos.

As with Yoga, there are many different types of Tai Chi to choose from. If you head to the Tai Chi Finder website - http://www.taichifinder.co.uk/classes - and click on your area, you will soon find a class.

CHAPTER FIFTY THREE:
TRAGER THERAPY.

Trager Therapy is a gentle method of movement education.

It was developed by Dr. Milton Trager, after 50 years of experience with the body, as a therapist and doctor.

The movements work to release unproductive physical and mental patterns to encourage deeper relaxation and increased motion. Trager bodyworks use light, gentle motions to release deep-seated physical and mental patterns which can be caused by poor posture, injuries, traumas, poor movement and stress.

It involves both table work and dance like movements. A session usually lasts from 60 – 90 minutes. No oils or lotions are used and the client is dressed for their comfort. The movements are never forced so that there is no induced pain or discomfort.

A good book on this therapy is *'Trager for Self Healing: A Practical Guide for Living in the Present Moment'*, by Audrey Mairi.

To find out more about Trager Therapy and to find a local practitioner head to this website - http://www.trager.com/approach.html

CHAPTER FIFTY FOUR
TRIGGER POINT THERAPY.

Chronic pain is often identified as arthritis, bursitis, carpal tunnel syndrome, sciatic symptoms, tendonitis, Angina Pectoris and Fibromyalgia.

In many cases, however, a misdiagnosis is involved, and the pain is actually caused by trigger points in the muscles. This can be diagnosed correctly and treated through trigger point massage therapy, given by professional massage therapists.

Dr. Janet G. Travell, personal physician of US President John F. Kennedy, discovered and mapped out trigger points in 1942. Trigger points are nodules that are contractions in bands of muscles that have tightened. The trigger points themselves cause local pain while simultaneously referring pain to other body parts.

The referred pain is often located far from the trigger point. Painful trigger points that actively refer pain to other body parts are called active trigger points.

Trigger point massage therapists identify a patient's trigger points and use deep prolonged pressure to deactivate then resolve them (a bit like acupressure). The therapist uses hands, fingers, knuckles, elbows, feet and many massage tools to apply and maintain such deep pressure consistently.

After resolving the trigger points, the therapist works further on the muscles and fascia, using their natural range of motion to stretch, elongate and relax them.

A great detailed book on the subject which I have found really useful is *'The Trigger Point Therapy Workbook: Your Self Treatment Guide for Pain Relief'*, by Clair Davies, Amber Davies and David G Simons.

It is dangerous to get trigger point massage therapy from an untrained therapist, though. Trigger points will not be resolved if not enough pressure is applied or if it is not held long enough. If too much pressure is applied, on the other hand, or if the pressure is held too long, the trigger point may be bruised and this will lead to even greater pain.

The untrained therapist may also cause the development of new trigger points or the activation of existing latent trigger points.

For more information, visit - http://www.myofascialtherapy.org/

CHAPTER FIFTY FIVE:
VIBRATION THERAPY.

Vibration Therapy is receiving a lot of attention at the moment, as it not only improves mobility in older people, but it can also help with the pain of Fibromyalgia and some types of Arthritis. It has also been incorporated into insoles to improve balance.

Vibration Therapy entails using a mechanical vibration machine to treat and prevent physical complaints including injuries and pain.

It is based on the scientific principle that all matter vibrates to a precise frequency and that by using resonant vibration, balance of matter can be restored.

Some researchers think that the vibration may over-ride pain signals going to the nervous system and thus leave you in less pain. It can also help with weight loss.

A good book on the subject is *'Raise Your Vibration, Transform Your Life: A Practical Guide for Attaining Better Health, Vitality and Inner Peace'*, by Dawn James and Andrea Lemieux.

A good website on this is - http://www.soundhealersassociation.org/dr-peter-guy-manners-vibrational-therapy

CHAPTER FIFTY SIX:
WATSU THERAPY.

Watsu massage is an underwater massage that takes place in warm, waist-deep water.

The weightlessness that the buoyancy of the water gives you, can be accompanied by a trained practitioner, known as watsuers, who will guide you into deep stretches in the pool of warm water.

A watsuer uses his or her own body to enhance the series of stretches that are being performed on the client, by bracing certain positions or wrapping the client's body around his or her own.

It was developed by Harold Dull back in 1980, and since that time its popularity has grown.

Dull, who had studied Zen Shiatsu in Japan, brought the principles of his Asian education back to North America where he was a massage therapist. He coined the idea of using the buoyancy of water to stretch his patient's bodies, improving the flow of their vital energy throughout their bodies.

Its name comes from a combination of the words 'water' and 'shiatsu'. It is also an excellent form of physical therapy for people with physical disabilities, such as arthritis, lower back pain, fibromyalgia, multiple sclerosis, spina bifida or paralysis.

It is also a great form of physical therapy for children, adults and seniors alike.

While for many people it takes just one Watsu session to become a believer, it may not be the right kind of massage therapy for everyone. That's because it requires an enormous amount of trust because, after all, you are putting yourself literally in the hands of another person for a full hour and you are both in the water. And, your eyes are closed!

Another good website on this type of treatment is Watsu Aqua Therapy UK at - http://www.watsuaquatherapy.co.uk/

CHAPTER FIFTY SEVEN:
YOGA.

Yoga is based on rhythm and breathing rather than core strength, so it's useful for relaxation and stress. There are lots of different types of Yoga available today but some good ones for pain are Bikram Yoga, Yin, Iyenger Yoga and Glow Yoga.

Bikram Yoga is a unique series of 26 Hatha Yoga postures and 2 breathing exercises, performed in a heated room to enhance your stretching.

It covers a series of postures which have been scientifically designed to work every part of the body in the correct order. The heat facilitates stretching, prevents injury and promotes sweating, which aids detoxification.

Yin Yoga is a yoga for the joints that stretches the connective tissue. It is a very distinctive style of Chinese yoga, which some believe is the oldest form of Hatha yoga.

Yang exercises work your heart and muscles and the exercises are floor-based. Lying down can immediately relax your body and unlike other Yogas, you hold your posture for up to ten minutes. It has been said to feel like 'peeling off layers of tension'.

Iyenger Yoga is perfect for people who feel 'stiff'. It's the safest and most effective way to stretch your whole body and improve your flexibility. It's characterised by great attention to detail and precise focus on body alignment with the use of 'props', such as cushions, benches, blocks and even sand bags. There are more than 200 deep poses, which you work towards holding for up to two minutes, which make it great for lengthening your muscles.

They say it is a perfect type of yoga, if you've got a muscular or joint injury.

With so many different types of Yoga available, it gets a bit confusing as to which one to choose, but it's really a case of try one, then try another.

Failing that, head to the British Wheel of Yoga website for more details at - http://www.bwy.org.uk/ - which claims to have the largest yoga community.

My book of choice would be *'Yoga Therapy: A Guide to the Therapeutic Use of Yoga and Ayurveda For Health and Fitness'*, by A G Mohan.

Postscript.

The author hopes you have found something of interest in the 57 alternative and complementary therapies briefly described in this book.

A bibliographic reference is included on each page where available, and naturally much of the information included in this book follows intensive research by Barbara on various internet search engines, for which permission to publish would be impossible to obtain.

The author would like to thank the creators of all sources of material to which she has referred here, however discovered.

If you require any further information, refer to Barbara's website at www.backpain.blog.co.uk or to the various books and websites given throughout.

Good luck with finding the treatment that helps you!

www.ingramcontent.com/pod-product-compliance
Lightning Source LLC
Chambersburg PA
CBHW070918180526
45168CB00005B/2055